Fatoumata FANE

Chemoprevention of seasonal malaria in children

AF546336

Fatoumata FANE

Chemoprevention of seasonal malaria in children

from 3 to 59 months in the Kati health district

ScienciaScripts

Imprint

Any brand names and product names mentioned in this book are subject to trademark, brand or patent protection and are trademarks or registered trademarks of their respective holders. The use of brand names, product names, common names, trade names, product descriptions etc. even without a particular marking in this work is in no way to be construed to mean that such names may be regarded as unrestricted in respect of trademark and brand protection legislation and could thus be used by anyone.

Cover image: www.ingimage.com

This book is a translation from the original published under ISBN 978-620-6-72191-8.

Publisher:
Sciencia Scripts
is a trademark of
Dodo Books Indian Ocean Ltd. and OmniScriptum S.R.L publishing group

120 High Road, East Finchley, London, N2 9ED, United Kingdom
Str. Armeneasca 28/1, office 1, Chisinau MD-2012, Republic of Moldova, Europe
Printed at: see last page
ISBN: 978-620-8-32578-7

Copyright © Fatoumata FANE
Copyright © 2024 Dodo Books Indian Ocean Ltd. and OmniScriptum S.R.L publishing group

DEDICATIONS AND THANKS

DEDICACES

❖ I give thanks to **ALLAH** the Almighty and Merciful for having enabled us to carry out this work and for having assisted us in all circumstances and in all places.

❖ To his Prophet **Mohamed,** may the peace and blessing of GOD be upon him, and to all his faithful companions.

❖ To my father, **Fané Oumar,** I really can't find the words to thank you most sincerely; you are the source of what I have become today. Your rigor, perseverance and courage in your work have been an inexhaustible source of inspiration for us. You surrounded us with attention, instilled in us the noble values of life, and taught us the meaning of work, honesty and responsibility. Thank you for always being there for me, a great support throughout my studies. You have always fought for the success of your children, and this modest work is the fruit of all the sacrifices you have made for my education and training.

❖ To my mother, **Dolo Kassatou**, you who gave me the breath of life, you who raised me in the serenity of the heart, you who nurtured and educated me, the most wonderful of all mothers. Your sense of generosity in everyday life has not left me indifferent. Time and again you sacrificed your own comforts just to please us. Your prayers and blessings have made it possible for me to brave the ups and downs of life without fear or worry.

ACKNOWLEDGEMENTS

❖ To all my teachers, from primary to secondary school, and to all the faculty of the Faculty of Pharmacy (FAPH), you have provided us with quality courses and instilled in us the quest for excellence. Thank you for all you have done for our training. May God reward you, and may you see in this work the fruits of the dedication you have shown during your teaching.

❖ To the staff of the Centre Hospitalier Universitaire Pr Bocar Sidy SALL de Kati, and in particular to those of the Pharmacie Hospitalière, I was warmly welcomed from my very first day, and felt right at home. Learning and working alongside you has been an immense pleasure.

❖ To the class of **the late Pr Drissa Diallo,** thank you for the many memories of the years we spent together. All these years spent together will remain among the best of my life, thanks to you. I would like you to know that I have a deep friendship with you.

❖ To **Dr. Nouhoun Diallo** and all the staff at the **BAZI GOURMA** pharmacy, thank you for your daily support and guidance, the spirit of teamwork, understanding and tolerance, especially at work.

❖ For fear of an unintentional omission, I would like to thank all those who have contributed in any way to the development of this thesis and to the success of this academic journey.

❖ I would like to thank the members of the jury for their presence, for their careful reading of this thesis, and for the comments and suggestions that helped me to bring this work to a successful conclusion.

TRIBUTE TO JURY MEMBERS

TO OUR MASTER AND PRESIDENT OF THE JURY

Pr Sanou Khô Coulibaly

- **Senior lecturer in toxicology at FMOS ;**
- **Specialist in Toxicology ;**
- **Lecturer in Toxicology at FMOS ;**
- **Expert in venimology ;**
- **Member of the African Society of Toxicology.**

Dear Master

You have done us a great honor by agreeing to chair this jury, despite your busy schedule. Your scientific rigor, your diligence, your approachability, your deep desire to enhance the profession make you a great man of science whose high scientific culture commands the respect and admiration of all.

It is a great honor and a source of pride for us to be among your students. Please accept our sincere thanks and the expression of our infinite gratitude.

TO OUR MASTER AND JUDGE

Dr Ismaïla SIMAGA

- **Chief Medical Officer of the Kati Health District ;**
- **Member of the group responsible for revising the management modules for community health centers ;**
- **Member of the commission responsible for implementing the new free services.**

Dear Master.

We are honored by your presence on this thesis jury. We were touched by your simplicity and availability. Your scientific, pedagogical and human culture, as well as your comments and suggestions, have greatly contributed to improving the quality of this work. Please accept, dear Master, the expression of our deepest gratitude and respect.

TO OUR MASTER AND JUDGE

Dr Sylvestre TRAORE

- **Pharmacist practitioner at the CHU Bocar Sidy SALL in Kati ;**
- **Pharmaceutical Management Assistant at FAPH ;**
- **Specialist in supply management and healthcare logistics.**

Dear Master

We were very honoured to have you as a member of our jury.

Your commitment to scientific research, your teaching skills, your dedication to a job well done and your perceptive analysis were all very useful to us in bringing this work to a successful conclusion.

Please accept, dear master, the expression of our deepest respect, our sincere gratitude and our best expressed thanks.

TO OUR MASTER AND CO-DIRECTOR

Dr Mohamed dit Sarmoye TRAORE

- **Specialist in Hospital Pharmacy at FAPH ;**
- **Head of the Hospital Pharmacy Department at CHU Pr Bocar Sidy SALL in Kati.**

Dear Master

It's an honor and a great pleasure for us to have you co-direct this work, of which you are in fact the instigator.

Throughout our career, you have instilled rigor in our work, and we have been fascinated by your sense of responsibility, your availability and your love of a job well done. Every exchange with you was an opportunity to enrich our knowledge. Dear Master, you have our deepest gratitude and appreciation.

TO OUR MASTER AND THESIS **DIRECTOR**

Pr Souleymane DAMA

- **Senior lecturer in Parasitology-Mycology at FAPH;**
- **Vice-dean of the FAPH Faculty of Pharmacy;**
- **Specialist in Preclinical and Clinical Pharmacology;**
- **Research teacher at FAPH.**

Dear Master

It is a great honor for you to accept the direction of this work. We have discovered in you a simple, enthusiastic and open-minded man who, despite his rank, erects no barriers with his students. These qualities make you an exceptional and exemplary person. Dear Master, please accept the expression of our deep respect and gratitude.

ACRONYMS AND ABBREVIATIONS

CHW: Community Health Worker

AQ: Amodiaquine

AN-RM: National Assembly of the Republic of Mali

ASACO: Community Health Association

AS: Artesunate

CPS: Chemoprevention of Seasonal Malaria

CSComs: Community Health Center

CSRéf: Centre de Santé de Référence

CHU-Gt: Gabriel Touré University Hospital

CHU-Point G: Point G University Hospital

GPRSP: Growth and Poverty Reduction Strategy Paper

MTEF: Medium-Term Expenditure Framework

ACT: Artemisinin-based Combination Therapy

MHC: Major Histocompatibility Complex

CSP: CircumSprorozoite Protein

DARC: Duffy Antigen Receptor for Chemokins

G6PD: Glucose-6-Phosphate Dehydrogenase

IL4: InterLeukine-4

INSP: Institut National du Service Public

NGO: Non-Governmental Organization

WHO: World Health Organization

PMA: Paquet Minimum d'Activité

PDDSS: Ten-Year Health and Social Development Plan

PRODESS: Socio-Sanitary Development Program

PNLP: National Malaria Control Program

PLDH: Parasite Lactate Dehydrogenase

SIS: Health Information System

SEC: Community Essential Care

SP: Sullfadoxine-Pyrimethamine

RDT: Rapid Diagnostic Test

T: Thymus

TNFα: Tumor Necrosis Factor α

SUMMARIES

INTRODUCTION 13
OBJECTIVES 15
General objective 15
Specific objectives 15
I. GENERAL 17
1.1 Historical background 17
1.2 Parasite cycle 18
1.3 Pathophysiology of malaria 21
1.4 Diagnosis of malaria 24
1.5 Treatment of malaria 27
1.6 Malaria prevention methods 29
II. METHODOLOGY 37
2.1 Setting and location of the study 37
2.2 Types of study 38
2.3 Collection period 38
2.4 Materials used 38
2.5 Data collection tools 38
4.6 Data entry and analysis 38
4.7 Data distribution authorization 38
III. RESULTS 40
IV. COMMENTS AND DISCUSSION 47
V. CONCLUSIONS AND RECOMMENDATIONS 51
VI. REFERENCES 54
IX. APPENDICES 58

INTRODUCTION

INTRODUCTION

Malaria is an infectious parasitic disease caused by the *Plasmodium* parasite, transmitted mainly by the bites of infected female Anopheles mosquitoes. Five species of Plasmodium are known to infect humans. These are : *Plasmodium falciparum* (*P. falciparum*), *Plasmodium malariae (P. malariae*), *Plasmodium vivax* (*P. vivax*), *Plasmodium ovale* (*P. ovale*) and *Plasmodium knowlesi* (*P. knowlesi*). Two of these five Plasmodium species responsible for human malaria are particularly dangerous. *Plasmodium falcifarum*, which causes the most deaths, is also the most widespread on the African continent. Then there's *Plasmodium vivax*, the dominant species in most countries outside sub-Saharan Africa. According to the World Health Organization's latest estimates, the number of malaria cases in 2023 will be 249 million, an increase of cases compared with 2021. The WHO African Region continues to bear a disproportionate share of the global malaria burden. In 2022, it accounted for 95% of global malaria morbidity and mortality. Children under the age of 5 accounted for around 80% of all malaria deaths in the region, making malaria a major cause of child mortality. [1]. With a view to eradicating malaria, the WHO, through its National Malaria Control Program (PNLP), has recommended a number of interventions to combat the disease. These include the use of Long-Acting Insecticide-Treated Nets (LLINs), indoor residual spraying of insecticides for vector control, rapid access to diagnostic tests when malaria is suspected, and treatment of confirmed cases. [2]. Despité these preventive measures, malaria remains a major concern in sub-Saharan Africa. This is why, in 2012, after numerous studies, the WHO recommended the implementation of a program to protect children under 5 years of age living in areas where malaria is endemic and transmission takes place mainly during a limited period, which is the rainy season. This new strategy is called Chemoprevention of Seasonal Malaria. It involves the use of drugs or drug combinations to prevent malaria infection and its consequences in the most vulnerable groups during the period of high transmission. [3].

In 2020, in Africa, the introduction of SPC led to a reduction in the number of malaria cases of over 65% in the intervention regions of Mali, and up to 86% in Chad [4]. However, according to data from the health information system, the number of malaria cases in children aged 3 to 59 months in the Kati health district continues to rise year on year [5]. These observations have led us to evaluate CPS data for children aged 3 to 59 months over the three-year period (2020-2021-2022) in the Kati health district, in order to analyze this trend.

OBJECTIVES

OBJECTIVES

General objective

To evaluate data from seasonal malaria chemoprevention (CPS) campaigns in children aged 3 to 59 months in the Kati health district.

Specific objectives

- ❖ Identify the reasons why children under the age of 5 who took part in the various campaigns did not take CPS medicines;
- ❖ Determine the coverage rates of the various SPC campaigns in the Kati health district;
- ❖ Verify the incidence of malaria in children under 5 in health facilities.

GENERAL

I. GENERAL

1.1 Historical background

Malaria is a very old disease, and it is thought that prehistoric man must have suffered from it. The disease probably originated in Africa, and followed human migrations along the Mediterranean coast to India and Southeast Asia. In the past, malaria was common in the Pontine marshes around Rome, and its name was derived from the Italian word for malaria or "bad air". It was also known as "Roman fever". The history of the disease can be considered on several levels: clinical, biological and therapeutic [6].

Clinically

The symptoms of intermittent fever were described by Hippocrates in the 5th century BC. He linked these fevers to certain climatic and environmental conditions, and divided them into three types according to their periodicity: daily, tierce or quarte. By the 2nd century B.C., the Greeks and Romans had already established a link between intermittent fevers and the proximity of swamps. Avicenna and Avenzoar described malarial splenomegaly and, after the Romans, considered the role of mosquitoes in malarial transmission [6].

Biologically speaking

In 1878, the malarial hematzoan was discovered by Alphonse Laveran, a French military physician, in Bône, Algeria (now Annaba), and confirmed in Constantine (Algeria) in 1880 by the observation of an ex flagellation. He demonstrated the parasitic nature of the condition by detecting the pathogenic agent in the blood of patients suffering from intermittent fever: *Plasmodium*.

From 1885 to 1897, in Italy, the work of Marchiafava, Celli, Golgi, Grassi, Welch and Fatelli confirmed the parasitic origin of the disease, and they discovered the first three species:

- *Plasmodium vivax* ;
- *Plasmodium falciparum* ;
- *Plasmodium malariae.*

In 1897, Ross, an Indian Army physician, proved the role of mosquitoes in the transmission of malaria.

In 1898, Grassi confirmed Ross's thesis and demonstrated that the female anopheles was the vector of the disease.

In 1922, Stephens described a fourth plasmodial species: *Plasmodium ovale.*

In 1930, Raffaele described exo-erythrocytic schizogony.

In 1948, Short and Garnham discovered the intrahepatic stage of parasite development in the human body.

A fifth species has recently been described (1965) in Southeast Asia: *Plasmodium knowlesi* [6].

Therapeutically

In 1630, Don Francisco Lopez learned from the Indians of Peru (South America) about the virtues of cinchona bark, the "fever tree".
In 1820, pharmacists Pierre Joseph Pelletier and Bienaimé Caventou isolated and chemically identified cinchona's active alkaloid: quinine.
In 1891, Erlich and Guttman observed the anti-plasmodial properties of Methylene Blue.
In 1926, the first synthetic antimalarial was obtained: Primaquine, an Amino-8-quinoline.
In 1934, Andersa synthesized Amino-4-quinoline derivatives including sentoquine and chloroquine.
In 1934, the synthesis of Amodiaquine, along with chloroquine, formed the basis of antimalarial therapy.
Curd et al. demonstrated the anti-malarial activity of certain biguanides, the first molecule synthesized being proguanil.
In 1961, the simultaneous emergence of chloroquine resistance in *P. falciparum* strains and insecticide resistance in Anopheles strains was noted.
From 1963 onwards, work focused on developing molecules active against chloroquine-resistant *Plasmodium* strains.
In 1971, this work led to the development of mefloquine and halofantrine.
In 1972, researchers at the Shanghai Institute, led by pharmacologist Youyou Tu, demonstrated the antiplasmodial activity of an extract of Artemisia annua L.(Asteracea): Artemisinin or Quinghaosu [6].

1.2 Parasite cycle

- **In Anopheles**

The parasite's vector and primary host is the female Anopheles mosquito. Young mosquitoes ingest the parasite for the first time when they feed on the blood (necessary for the female to produce eggs) of an infected human subject. Once ingested, *Plasmodium* gametocytes differentiate into male and female gametes, then unite to form a mobile zygote, called an ookinete, which penetrates the mosquito's stomach wall to become a spherical oocyst, whose nucleus divides multiple times to form sporozoites. The duration of this maturation process is highly dependent on external temperature. For example, in the case of *P. falciparum*, maturation does not occur below 18°C or above 35°C, but is maximal at around 24°C. When the oocyst ruptures, it releases sporozoites which migrate through the mosquito's body to the salivary glands, from where they can infect a new human host during a new blood meal, passing through the skin with the saliva [7].

❖ **In humans**

Liver phase

A slender spindle measuring 12 µm / 1 µm, the infectious sporozoite injected into a human during a bite by an infected female Anopheles mosquito circulates rapidly (less than half an hour) through the bloodstream to the liver, where it is largely sequestered by the adhesive motifs of its major envelope protein, the circumsporozoite protein or CSP = Circumsporozoite protein, and then infects the hepatocytes. This hepatic pre-erythrocytic crisis, which lasts 7 to 15 days for *P. falciparum*, 15 days to 9 months for *P. vivax*, 15 days to X months for *P. ovale* and 3 weeks for *P. malariae*, enables the parasite to continue its cycle. Sporozoites that do not reach the liver are either eliminated by phagocytes, or are unable to continue their evolution if they reach other organs. A first transformation rounds off this "cryptozoite" form (from the Greek kruptós, "hidden") into a uninucleated element (with a single nucleus) called a trophozoite, which gives the parasite the opportunity to multiply directly (this is always the case for *P. falciparum*), by schizogony, for a week to two weeks, culminating in an enormous schizont (the name given to the protozoan when it becomes active after the incubation phase) of 40 to 80 µm. This blue body (because it is made up of pale blue cytoplasm when stained with May-Grünwald-Giemsa) buds, while losing its mobility, so as to emit vesicles, containing the young merozoites that will be transferred to the blood, thus initiating the erythrocytic stage, i.e. infection of the red blood cells. However, some *P. ovale* or *P. vivax* merozoites can remain hidden in the liver for several years, or even a lifetime in the case of *P. malariae*, before reactivating in successive waves. These secondary exo-erythrocytic cycles maintain the parasite in the liver for two or three years in the case of *P. ovale*, 3 to 5 years or more in the case of *P. vivax*, and for life in the case of *P. malariae*. This phase of the parasite is known as the "dormant phase". These intra-hepatic latent parasites are called "hypnozoites" (from the Greek húpnos, "sleep") [7].

Transfer phase

The vesicles are released into the hepatic sinusoids (capillary vessels linking the liver to the bloodstream), where they enter the bloodstream and spread a stream of young "pre-erythrocytic" merozoites ready to infect red blood cells. Each infected liver cell contains around 100,000 merozoites (each schizont is capable of producing 20,000 merozoites). A true "Trojan Horse" technique is used here to move from liver cells to blood. In 2005-2006, in vivo imaging in rodents showed that merozoites were able to manufacture dead cells enabling them to leave the liver for the bloodstream, thus evading the immune system.) They seem to both guide this "vehicle" and hide within it, masking the biochemical signals that normally alert macrophages. This may be a new avenue for active drugs or an anti-exo-erythrocytic stage vaccine before the red blood cell invasion stage [7].

Blood phase

At the start of the long blood phase: merozoites attach to red blood cells, invade them, develop into trophozoites and then divide (schizonts).

In 2011, an international team discovered that one of the receptors on the surface of the red blood cell (confirmed with all *P. falciparum* strains tested) is essential for parasite entry, making it a target for future vaccine research. As they spread, merozoites burst red blood cells (hemolysis).

The bursting of mature schizonts or "rosettes" completes the first erythrocytic schizogonic cycle, releasing into the bloodstream a new generation of plasmodiums, the "erythrocytic" merozoites capable of reinfecting other red blood cells.

A regular succession of similar cycles will follow, gradually replaced (as immune defenses become organized) by gamogonous erythrocytic cycles in preparation for sexual forms. Trophozoites stop dividing and change their nucleoplasmatic ratio. These trophozoite forms, with their enlarged nuclei and denser cytoplasm, are male and female gametocytes, waiting in the blood.

During this phase, parasites have no chance of survival in humans: they remain alive for around twenty days, then disappear. They can only continue their evolution in mosquitoes. At this point, if a female Anopheles bites a sick person, it absorbs gametocytes from the blood, and a new cycle, this time sexual, begins in the mosquito. The sporozoites produced by this reproduction pass into the mosquito's saliva, which can then infect a new host, and so on [7].

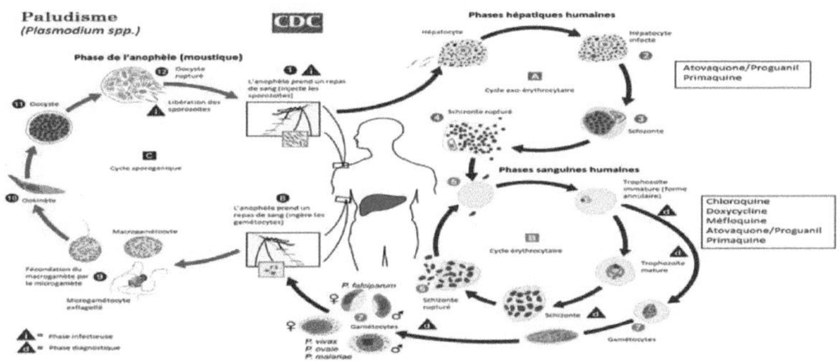

Figure 1 Life cycle of the parasite that causes malaria and main sites of drug activity [7].

1.3 Pathophysiology of malaria

Clinical manifestation

Hematozoa inoculated by the mosquito first localize and multiply in the liver. This phase defines a minimal incubation period, with no symptoms. Clinical manifestations of malaria appear at the start of the blood phase, when parasitaemia exceeds a threshold that varies from one individual to another. This asexual multiplication of Plasmodium inside red blood cells makes malaria, in the truest sense of the word, a parasitic disease of the red blood cells. Lysis of parasitized red blood cells (bursting of mature schizonts or rosettes) releases new parasites (merozoites), which in turn contaminate other red blood cells. This destruction also leads to the release of waste products from plasmodial metabolism (pigments and cellular debris from the red blood cell, or hemozoin). These pyrogenic substances disrupt the hypothalamus (production of cytokines such as TNFα) and cause high fevers. The first cycles are initially asynchronous (primo-invasion malaria, with continuous or anarchic fever), then they synchronize according to a periodic rhythm, depending on the *Plasmodium* species. The time elapsing between the penetration of a parasite into a red blood cell and its bursting is fairly constant, reaching 48 hours in humans for *P. vivax, P. ovale and P. falciparum* (third-grade fevers), 72 hours for *P. malariae* (fourth-grade fever); and only 24 hours for *P. knowlesi*, the latest species confirmed in humans. In cases of intense parasitization, red blood cells are destroyed to such an extent that hemolytic anemia and jaundice occur. The body reacts by hyperplasia (increased production) of macrophages, which explains the enlargement of the liver (hepatomegaly) and spleen (splenomegaly). *P. falciparum* differs from other

Plasmodium species in its ability to enter the bloodstream through visceral capillaries, particularly in brain tissue. This can lead to the formation of "rosettes" (clusters of healthy and parasitized red blood cells), which adhere to the capillary walls. This situation may be accompanied by secondary hypoxia, metabolic and hydro-electrolytic disturbances, and vascular (small vessel walls) and tissue lesions. If left untreated, *P. falciparum* malaria presents an immediate vital risk (e.g., risk of multi-visceral failure syndrome). The various forms of malaria are likely to evolve into chronic forms (historical forms), with progressive deterioration in general condition leading to cachexia [8].

Immunity

After several years of repeated infection, the Plasmodium host can acquire immunity, known as premunition (attenuated symptoms of a disease that protect against a later, more severe infection). Responses to malaria infection vary widely between individuals living in the same endemic areas. In regions where transmission is high, a large proportion of children are often carriers of *P. falciparum* parasites without reporting any symptoms; this is known as clinical immunity. With age and successive human/parasite contacts, this premunition gradually takes hold, calling on mechanisms of resistance to infection, among which the "interferon" proteins metabolized and excreted, among others, by the liver play a major role in anti-parasite immunity. This is known as tolerance to infection or anti-parasite immunity. One hypothesis is that *Plasmodium* needs iron to develop; iron deficiency due to a first infection would provide relative protection and avoid "superinfection". It is often said that this immunity is not sterilizing, as it has never been formally demonstrated that *P. falciparum* parasites disappear completely in the absence of treatment. This immunity is also said to be labile, as premunition disappears in the absence of frequent contact between humans and the parasite (it disappears after 12 to 24 months if the subject leaves the endemic zone), as well as in pregnant women. Furthermore, immunity to *P. falciparum* is highly specific to the parasite strain(s) present. These particularities of the immune response against malaria are at the root of the difficulties in developing a vaccine [8].

Genetic factor

Genetic factors can protect against malaria. Most of those described are associated with red blood cells. Here are a few examples:

- Sickle cell disease (from the Greek drepanos, meaning "sickle" in reference to the elongated shape of a certain number of red blood cells), also known as hemoglobinosis

S, sickle cell disease or sickle cell anemia: a change in the ß chain of hemoglobin deforms the red blood cells, producing heterozygotes with better protection against malaria. The red blood cells are deformed and the hemoglobin crystallizes, preventing the parasite from entering the red blood cell. However, this change leads to poor oxygenation of the organs (elongated red blood cells cannot pass through the fine capillaries or the spleen filter barrier, where they are destroyed) and, consequently, to severe complications, up to and including death in homozygous subjects (HbS/HbS). The prevalence of sickle cell disease (HbA/HbS) is high in African populations under heavy malaria pressure, due to the resistance it provides against severe bouts of the disease,

- Thalassemia or hereditary anemia: the subject carries the SS gene, which causes a change in the rate of synthesis of globin chains, resulting in poor blood circulation and constant fatigue,
- Genetic deficiency of G6PD (Glucose-6-phosphate dehydrogenase), also known as favism, an antioxidant enzyme that normally protects against the effects of oxidative stress in red blood cells, provides increased protection against severe malaria,
- HLA-B53 is associated with a low risk of severe malaria. This MHC (major histocompatibility complex) class I molecule, present in the liver, is an antigen of T lymphocytes (located in the thymus) against the sporozoite stage. This antigen, encoded by IL4 (Interleukin-4), produced by T cells (thymus), promotes the proliferation and differentiation of B-cell antibody production. A study of Fulani people in Burkina Faso, who have fewer than two malaria attacks with higher levels of anti-malarial antibodies than neighboring ethnic groups, found that the IL4-524 T allele was associated with high levels of anti-malarial antibodies, raising the possibility that it could be a factor in increasing resistance to malaria ;
- In the natural fight against *P. vivax* in Africa, the selection process has led to the disappearance from the genetic heritage of a membrane receptor on erythrocytes, the glycoprotein DARC (Duffy Antigen Receptor for Chemokines), which is the entry target for *P. vivax*. This means that subjects with a negative Duffy blood group, abbreviated FY (-), cannot be infected by *P. vivax*. This explains the absence of *P. vivax* in the West African population, which is exclusively or predominantly of the "Duffy-negative" blood group. However, this natural immunity could be called into question, as *P. vivax* has succeeded in adapting to Madagascar in Duffy-negative

subjects, as a result of genetic mixing between African and Asian populations. This would point to the existence of secondary targets for the parasite, yet to be determined.

Other genetic factors exist, some of which are involved in controlling the immune response [8].

1.4 Diagnosis of malaria

Clinical diagnosis

The initial symptoms of malaria (such as fever, chills, sweating, headaches, muscle aches, nausea and vomiting) are often non-specific and may also be associated with other illnesses (e.g. influenza and other viral infections). Similarly, clinical signs are often not explicit (high temperature, sweating and fatigue). However, in the case of severe malaria (mainly caused by *P. falciparum*), clinical features such as confusion, coma, convulsions, severe anemia, respiratory distress, are more precise and increase the index of suspicion of malaria [9].

Diagnosis

In all cases where malaria is suspected, the healthcare provider should carry out an initial work-up and arrange for a parasitological test, either by means of a quality-assured rapid diagnostic test (RDT), or by microscopic examination of a blood smear slide. One or both of these tests can be used as the main diagnostic tool for the confirmation and management of suspected clinical malaria, in any epidemiological situation, including areas of low transmission. For microscopic diagnosis, the thick drop is a more sensitive test for detecting the malaria parasite, while the smear enables better identification of the parasite species.

In addition, a blood test, including a complete blood count and routine chemistry, should be performed. If the malaria test is positive, these additional tests will be useful in determining whether the patient has simple or severe manifestations of the infection. These tests can detect severe anemia, hypoglycemia, renal failure, hyperbilirubinemia and acid-base disorders [9].

Techniques for using malaria diagnostic tests

Blood smear

- Place a drop of blood (approx. 5ul) on the tip of a slide;
- Using a second blade held at a 45-degree angle to the first, touch the drop of blood to the first blade, then break it off with a brief movement to obtain a fine spread;
- Dry immediately by shaking the blade;
- Fix the smear by covering the preparation with methanol at 95 degrees;
- Then tilt the blade to remove excess liquid and allow to dry completely;
- May-Grünwald-Giemsa (MGG) or Giemsa staining after fixation ;

- Observe with an optical microscope using an immersion 100 objective;
- The morphology of the parasites inside the red blood cells helps determine the species involved;
- Parasitemia can be estimated as a percentage of parasitized red blood cells.

The thin smear is a technique for the morphological study of haematozoa. Differential diagnosis between plasmodial species remains a challenge even for the trained reader. The sensitivity of the thin smear is between 100-200 parasitized red blood cells/ul; 50 parasites per ul [10].

Thick drop

- Place a drop of about 10ul of blood on a slide;
- Spread the drop over a diameter of 1cm, using a counter-clockwise circular motion for a few seconds;
- Allow to dry carefully (away from dust and flies). After drying, stain the slide with a 10% solution of Giemsa for 15 minutes;
- Rinse with distilled water and dry the slide thoroughly;
- Apply a drop of immersion oil and observe under a light microscope with objective 100 ;
- The leukocytes will appear with dark purple nuclei and the parasite will show dark red chromatin with pale blue cytoplasm;
- The number of parasites is counted on 200 leukocytes, and the average number of leukocytes/blood unit is estimated at 8,000.

Parasitemia is calculated using the following formula: Number of parasites counted x 8000/200 = parasitemia per ul of blood.

The sensitivity of the thick drop is 5-10 parasites/blood unit. [10].

Rapid tests for parasitic antigens

They are an aid to diagnosis, but do not replace the smear and thick drop.

- **HRP II antigen**

HRP II is a glycoprotein plasmodial antigen. It appears on the surface of red blood cells specifically parasitized by *Plasmodium falciparum*, and is secreted during the intra-erythrocytic cycle, peaking at schizont rupture. Only asexual forms of *P. falciparum* express this glycoprotein. Tests for its detection are based on the principle of immuno-chromatography. This soluble protein was the first to be used in rapid diagnostic tests. At least five malaria proteins (HRP I, HRP II, EMP I, EMP II, and EMP III) have been identified in the surface or in association with the cytoskeleton of *Plasmodium falciparum-infected* erythrocytes. HRPII is a histidine- and alanine-rich protein localized in several cellular compartments, including the parasite cytoplasm. The content of histidine (H), alanine (A) and aspartic acid (D) in HRPII is 34%, 10% and 10% respectively. It is characterized by several contiguous repeats of the AHH and AHHAAD orders. Histidine-rich proteins were among the first plasmodial proteins to be studied in detail. They were first isolated from cytoplasmic inclusions in the asexual stages of *P. lophurae*, a malaria parasite. To date, the exact function of HRPII is not well understood. The histidine-rich protein II of *P. falciparum* has been identified as a heme polymerase that detoxifies free heme by polymerization to inactive hemozoans. It has been shown to be a hexapeptide repeat (Ala-His-His-AlaAla-Asp) that appears 33 times in Pf HRP II, and may be the main acceptor of heme. Currently, the main application of detailed knowledge of HRPII is its use in malaria diagnosis by detection of P. falciparum HRPII antigen. There is a prolonged circulation of HRPII, detectable a fortnight after the parasites have disappeared from the circulating blood. This longer clearance of HRPII allows retrospective diagnosis of the presence of *P. falciparum*, but does not allow us to judge the efficacy of anti-malarial treatment. Detection by immuno-chromatography on whole blood takes less than 10 minutes, with a specificity of around 90%. Sensitivity ranges from 83% to 100%, as the test may be compromised by low parasitaemia, association with *P. vivax* or a high proportion of gametocytes [11].

PLDH antigen

The intraerythrocytic stage of *Plasmodium falciparum* depends mainly on the energy generated by glycolysis. The NAD consumed during glycolysis is regenerated by pyruvate fermentation in the cell cytoplasm and/or by the electron transport chain in the mitochondria. Unlike mammalian cells and most aerobic organisms, lactate is the final product of the glycolytic pathway *in Plasmodium*. Lactate dehydrogenase (LDH) catalyzes the reduction of pyruvate to lactate in the presence of NADH. This enables rapid energy production according to the parasite's requirements. pLDH has now been identified, and specific inhibition of this enzyme represents a potential target for anti-malarial therapeutic molecules. The pLDH enzyme is produced by all human parasites during their intraerythrocytic development. The detection of parasite lactate dehydrogenase (pLDH) was originally developed as a method of measuring parasite growth in vitro during drug susceptibility testing. The principle of the test is that the parasite enzyme (pLDH) has different biochemical characteristics to human LDH and can, therefore, be measured differentially using a simple colorimetric assay [12].

Aldolase

Other enzymes involved in the glycolytic pathway of *Plasmodium* have been recognized and considered as targets for rapid diagnostic tests. Since citric acid is absent during energy metabolism in the endo-erythrocytic phase of *Plasmodium*, ATP production depends entirely on glycolysis; Aldolase is a key enzyme in this pathway. In experiments to determine the stage of Aldolase production, it was shown that this enzyme is made up of two isoenzymes: aldo-1, which is specific to *Plasmodium falciparum*, and aldo-2, found in *Plasmodium* species other than *P. falciparum*. Monoclonal antibodies used to detect Aldolase are non-specific. Used in rapid tests, they are usually combined with HRP II to detect both *Plasmodium falciparum* and *Plasmodium vivax*. It is detected in the parasite membrane and in the cytoplasm of the host red blood cell. [12].

1.5 Treatment of malaria

Malaria is a preventable and curable disease. The primary aim of treatment is to achieve complete cure, i.e. the rapid and total elimination of malaria parasites from the patient's bloodstream, to prevent uncomplicated malaria from progressing to a severe, potentially fatal form, or to a chronic infection causing anemia. From a public health point of view, the aim of treatment is to reduce transmission of the infection by reducing the infectious reservoir, and to prevent the emergence and spread of resistance to antimalarial drugs [13].

The importance of diagnostic tests

For all patients suspected of having malaria, parasitological confirmation of the diagnosis should be obtained by microscopic examination or a rapid diagnostic test before treatment is started. Treatment should only be administered on the basis of clinical examination if diagnostic tests cannot be carried out within 2 hours of consultation. Prompt treatment, within 24 hours of the onset of fever, with a safe and effective antimalarial is essential to enable recovery and avoid life-threatening complications [13].

Treatment of uncomplicated malaria

- **Treatment of P. falciparum infections**

The WHO recommends artemisinin-based combination therapies (ACTs) to treat uncomplicated malaria caused by *P. falciparum*. Combining 2 active ingredients with different modes of action, ACTs are the most effective antimalarial drugs available today. The WHO currently recommends 5 ACTs against *P. falciparum* malaria. The choice of ACTs should be based on the results of therapeutic efficacy studies against local strains *of P. falciparum* malaria. ACTs form the backbone of the recommended treatment against *P. falciparum* malaria, and since no other artemisinin derivative is expected to be marketed for several years, their efficacy must be preserved. WHO recommends that national malaria control programs regularly monitor the efficacy of antimalarial drugs in use, to ensure that the treatments chosen remain effective. In low-transmission areas, a single dose of primaquine should be added to antimalarial treatment to reduce transmission of infection. Screening for glucose-6-phosphate dehydrogenase (G6PD) deficiency is not necessary, as a low single dose of primaquine is both effective in blocking transmission and unlikely to have toxic effects in G6PD-deficient subjects, regardless of the genotypic variants involved [13].

- **Oral monotherapy and artemisinin resistance**

Artemisinin and its derivatives should not be used as oral monotherapy, as this encourages the development of artemisinin resistance. In addition, fixed-dose combinations (combining 2 different active ingredients in a single tablet) are clearly preferable and strongly recommended to blister, single-pack or bulk combinations, as they facilitate compliance and limit the risk of tablets being used separately as monotherapy. [13].

- **Treatment of P. vivax infections**

P. vivax infections should be treated with either ACT or chloroquine in areas where chloroquine resistance does not exist. In areas where chloroquine-resistant strains *of P. vivax* have been identified, infections should be treated with an ACT, preferably a combination in which the drug associated with artemisinin has a long half-life. With the exception of artesunate + sulfadoxine- pyrimethamine (AS+SP), all ACTs are effective against blood-stage *P. vivax* infections. In order to prevent relapses, primaquine should be added to treatment; dosage and frequency of administration will need to be adjusted according to each patient's glucose-6-phosphate dehydrogenase (G6PD) enzymatic activity [13].

Treatment of severe malaria

Severe malaria should be treated with injectable artesunate (intramuscular or intravenous) for at least 24 hours, followed by a full 3-day course of ACT once the patient can tolerate oral medication. When injectable treatment cannot be administered, children under 6 years of age with severe malaria should receive rectal artesunate before being referred immediately to a center capable of providing full parenteral treatment. It is imperative that artemisinin-based injectable treatments and artesunate-based suppositories are not used as monotherapy. Initial treatment of severe malaria with these drugs must be supplemented by a full 3-day course of ACT. This ensures complete cure and prevents the development of resistance to artemisinin derivatives [13].

1.6 Malaria prevention methods

Reducing human-vector contact

Malaria can be prevented by avoiding mosquito bites and taking medication. Consult a doctor to find out if you can take chemo-prophylactic drugs before traveling to areas where malaria is common.

Limit the risk of contracting malaria by avoiding mosquito bites:

- ❖ Use mosquito nets when sleeping in places where malaria is present;
- ❖ Use of mosquito repellents after dusk ;
- ❖ Use of mosquito sprays or sprays;
- ❖ Wearing protective clothing ;
- ❖ Vaccination ;
- ❖ Placing insect screens on windows [14].

Intermittent preventive treatment for pregnant women

Intermittent preventive treatment should be administered to all pregnant women from the beginning of the second trimester. It reduces episodes of malaria in the mother and the associated risks. SP meets WHO expectations for intermittent preventive treatment. It should be used during the second and third trimesters of pregnancy.

The usual dosage is three tablets taken in a single dose three times during pregnancy. The first dose during the second trimester and the second dose during the third trimester of pregnancy. In some cases, your doctor may recommend a third dose. The last dose should be taken at least thirty days before the due date. [14]. **1.6.1 Chemoprevention of Seasonal Malaria (CPS)**

It is recommended in areas of high seasonal malaria transmission throughout the Sahel region. Its strategy is to administer a complete course of **Amodiaquine** and **Sullfadoxine-Pyrimethamine** (AQ-SP) in children aged 3 to 59 months at regular one-month intervals, starting at the beginning of the transmission season and giving a maximum of four doses during it (provided that both drugs retain sufficient antimalarial efficacy). [15].

CPS objectives

The main objective is to contribute to :

- ❖ Reduce the number of cases of simple or severe malaria ;
- ❖ Reduce the number of hospitalizations due to malaria;
- ❖ Reducing malaria morbidity and mortality in children under 5.

The specific objective is to maintain therapeutic concentrations of antimalarial drugs in the blood during the period when the risk of malaria is highest. [16].

Choice of Sullfadoxine-Pyrimethamine and Amodiaquine

The SP+AQ association was chosen by CPS for the following reasons:

❖ Clinical trials have shown that the combination of MS+AQ confers better protection than other drug combinations. The use of both drugs in dual therapy limits the risk of selecting resistance to MS or AQ as monotherapy;

❖ SP and AQ retain their therapeutic efficacy in Sahelian and Sub-Sahelian zones of seasonal transmission where SPC is appropriate;

❖ MS+AQ treatment is well tolerated and relatively inexpensive;

❖ SP+AQ combination does not contain **artemisinin** derivatives [17].

Drug characteristics (AQ -SP)

They are all in tablet form, so oral administration is difficult in children and infants.

❖ **Sullfadoxine-Pyrimethamine** is a combination of a sulfonamide and an anti-folinic Diamino pyrimidine. It is also an endo-erythrocytic schizonticide, but slow-acting. The duration of action and plasma half-life is around 9 hours. [17].

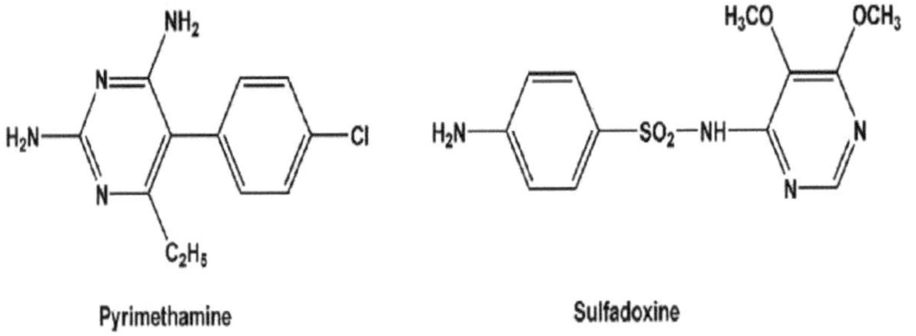

Pyrimethamine Sulfadoxine

Figure 2 Chemical structure of Sullfadoxine-Pyrimethamine (www.researchgate.net)

❖ **Amodiaquine**, a member of the amino-4-quinoline family, is a fast-acting endo-erythrocytic schizonticide with a duration of action and plasma half-life of approximately 10 to 30 days. [17].

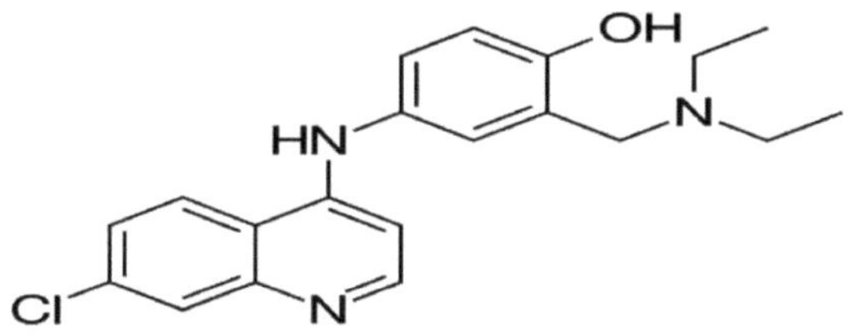

Figure 3Chemical structure of Amodiaquine (www.Amodiaquine.svg)

Drug storage

Medicines should be stored in a dry environment at a temperature of between 8 and 28 degrees, away from humidity and direct sunlight.

Recommended dosage according to age

- Infants <12 months: AQ-half of a 153 mg tablet once a day for three days and a single dose of SP-half of a 500/25 mg tablet.
- Children 12-59 months: AQ one whole tablet at 153 mg once a day for three days and a single dose of SP - one whole tablet at 500/25 mg.
- The single dose of SP is administered only on the first day with the first dose of AQ.
- Regardless of the child's age, the dosage should correspond to ½ SP tablet per 10kg as a single dose and 10mg/kg per day for three days. [18].

CPS indications

- Be in the hyperendemic zone during the prevention campaign;
- Children aged 3 to 59 months without confirmed malaria ;
- Children with no history of allergy to SP or AQ ;
- Child who has not received an antimalarial containing SP or AQ in the last 30 days;
- Children with no acute illness who are not receiving co-trimoxazole prophylaxis [18].

CPS contraindication

It should not be administered to :

- A child with a serious acute illness or unable to take oral medication;
- An HIV-positive child taking co-trimoxazole;
- A child who has had a dose of SP or AQ in the previous month;
- A child allergic to any of these drugs (SP-AQ) [18].

Target period for CPS

CPS must be carried out during the period of high transmission. The start and end dates depend on the pattern of malaria transmission, which is generally correlated with rainfall. Rainfall patterns differ from country to country and within countries. If the plan calls for the administration of three cycles of SPC treatment during the season of high malaria transmission, the second cycle should coincide with the peak of the transmission season.

Depending on the date of administration of the first treatment dose, the second, third and fourth cycles (if applicable) should follow at one-month intervals.

First cycle (first month)

- Day 0: single dose of SP + first dose of amodiaquine (by a health worker)
- Day 1: second dose of amodiaquine (parent or guardian)
- Day 2: third dose of amodiaquine (parent or guardian)

Second cycle (second month)

- Day 0: single dose of SP + first dose of amodiaquine (by a health worker)
- Day 1: second dose of amodiaquine (parent or guardian)
- Day 2: third dose of amodiaquine (parent or guardian)

Third cycle (third month)

- Day 0: single dose of SP + first dose of amodiaquine (by a health worker)
- Day 1: second dose of amodiaquine (parent or guardian)
- Day 2: third dose of amodiaquine (parent or guardian)

Fourth cycle (fourth month) if applicable

- Day 0: single dose of SP + first dose of amodiaquine (by a health worker)
- Day 1: second dose of amodiaquine (parent or guardian)
- Day 2: third dose of amodiaquine (parent or guardian)

The aim is to administer complete 3-day treatment cycles of SP + AQ to every eligible child at least three times during the period of high malaria transmission. Protection against clinical malaria is associated with the administration of the second and third doses of amodiaquine. Therefore, it is important that a child receives full doses of SP + AQ during each SPC treatment cycle. A maximum of four treatment cycles can be administered, depending on the malaria transmission profile. If a child misses a cycle of SPC treatment because he or she is sick or absent, he or she should receive the next cycle's drugs if present and well [17].

Side effects of SPC drugs [19].

QA side effects

Table I Minor QA events

Molecules	Minor events	Case definitions	What to do
Amodiaquine	Pruritus	Itching	Stop treatment and take antihistamine
	Digestive disorders	Nausea Vomiting Diarrhea anorexia Abdominal pain	Stop treatment Anti-emetics
	Skin rash	Skin rash	Discontinuation of treatment and antihistamines
	Headache	Headaches	Paracetamol
	Slate pigmentation		Stopping treatment
	Weakness	General fatigue	Monitoring
	Trembling		Monitoring
	Malaise	Headache	Monitoring
	Skin manifestations	Localized skin detachment (Lyell syndrome)	Stopping treatment
	Cardiac manifestations	Palpitation	Stopping treatment

Table II Serious QA events

	Serious events	Case definitions	What to do
Amodiaquine	Ocular manifestations: accommodation disorder; corneal opacification; conjunctival hyperemia	Blurred vision White spot on cornea Irritation	Stopping treatment
	Severe jaundice	Yellow coloring of integuments	Stopping treatment
	Skin manifestations	Localized skin detachment (Lyell syndrome)	Stopping treatment
	Severe anemia	Pale teguments	Stopping treatment
	Cardiac manifestations	Palpitation	Stopping treatment

Side effects of MS

Table III Minor symptoms of MS

Molecule	Minor events	Case definitions	What to do
Sullfadoxine-Pyrimethamine	Pruritus	Itching	Stop treatment and take antihistamine
	Digestive disorders	Nausea Vomiting Diarrhea anorexia Abdominal pain	Stop treatment Anti-emetics
	Skin rash	Skin rash	Discontinuation of treatment and antihistamines

Table IV Serious symptoms of MS

Molecule	Serious events	Case definitions	What to do
Sullfadoxine-Pyrimethamine	Agranulocytosis		Stopping treatment
	Thrombocytopenia		Stopping treatment
	Hepatic toxicity	Yellow coloring of integuments	Stopping treatment
	Purpura Thrombopenicus		Stopping treatment
	Granulocytopenia		Stopping treatment
	Severe anemia	Pale teguments	Stopping treatment
	Stevens-Johson syndrome		Stopping treatment
	Lyell syndrome		Stopping treatment

Advantages of CPS

The WHO strategic recommendation for SPC is based on the results of seven studies carried out in areas of high seasonal malaria transmission in the Sahelian and sub-Sahelian regions of sub-Saharan Africa. These studies show that SPC with monthly administration of SP + AQ in children aged 3 to 59 months for up to four months during the season of high malaria transmission:

- ❖ Avoids around 75% of all malaria attacks;
- ❖ Avoids about 75% of severe malaria attacks;
- ❖ Could lead to a reduction in infant mortality;
- ❖ Probably reduces the incidence of moderate anemia;
- ❖ Does not lead to a recrudescence of malaria exceeding the pre-CPS level during the following transmission season, one year after CPS administration;
- ❖ There have been no reports of serious adverse events, which are probably rare [20].

METHODOLOGY

II. METHODOLOGY

2.1 Scope and location of study

Our study took place in the Kati health district. From a historical point of view, the creation of the cercle de Kati is legendary and confused. According to stories told in the villages of M'PIEBOUGOU and BAMANANKIN (Kati Koro). According to these tales, shortly after the creation of KOKOBOUGOUNI by DJIEGNOUMA KOLEBA, an unsocial and stern family member (a KATIGUELEN) left the village to settle on the present-day site of Kati Koro. In 1880, a French troop commanded by Lieutenant GALIENI arrived in Kati, and in 1886 the Kati military camp was created and renamed Camp GALIENI de Kati. The Kati area covers a surface area of 9636 Km^2 and is bounded to the north by the cercle of Kolokani; to the east by the Cercle of Koulikoro; to the west by the Cercle of Kita; to the south by the health district of Kalaban Coro; to the south/west by the cercle of Kangaba and the Republic of Guinea-Conakry. The district of Bamako is embedded in that of Kati. From a health point of view, from its creation to 2022, the district of Kati had 44 CSComs. The population was estimated at 750,595 in 2022. The Centre de Santé de Références de Kati (CSRéf) is organized into sections and units divided into blocks.

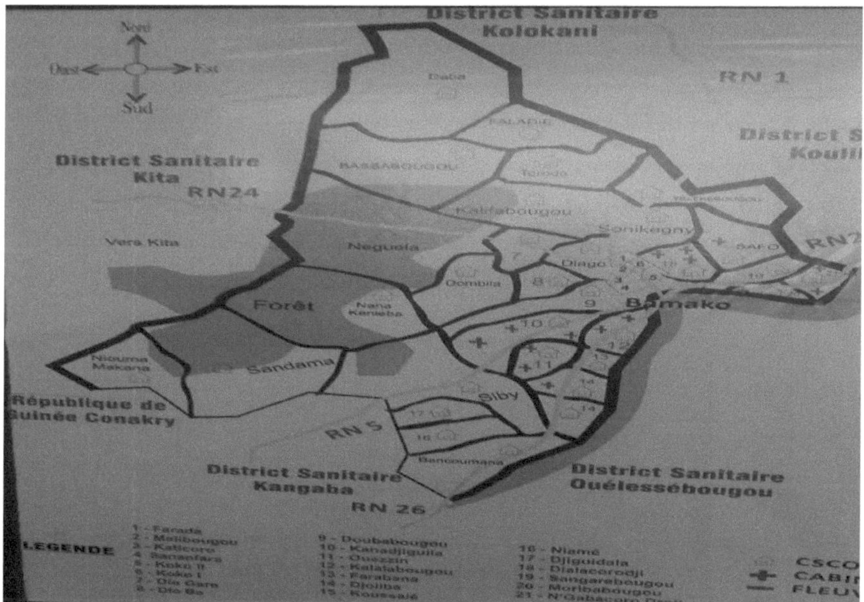

Figure 4:Map of the Kati health district [5].

2.2 Types of study

This is a retrospective, quantitative, cross-sectional study.

2.3 Collection period

Data collection took place over a three-month period from January 1 to March 31, 2023. It involved data from the various CPSs from January 1, 2020 to December 31, 2022 in the Kati health district.

2.4 Materials used

The material consisted of the reports of the 4 CPS passages of each year.

2.5 Data collection tools

Data collection was carried out by consulting the reports of the 4 CPS passages of each year. The data collected concerned :

- Number of children expected ;
- Age group concerned ;
- Sex;
- The various CSComs concerned.

4.6 Data entry and analysis

Data analysis was performed using Microsoft Excel 2013.

The CPS coverage rate was calculated using the following formula:

CPS coverage rate= (NECPS ×100)/NET

NECPS: Number of children having benefited from CPS in a given health area.

NET: Total number of children expected in a given health area

4.7 Data distribution authorization

The agreement of the Chief Medical Officer of the Kati CSRéf has been obtained to collect and evaluate data from the Kati CPS during the period from 2020 to 2022.

RESULTS

III. RESULTS

3.1 Number of children with a positive RDT compared to those who underwent RDT during SPCs

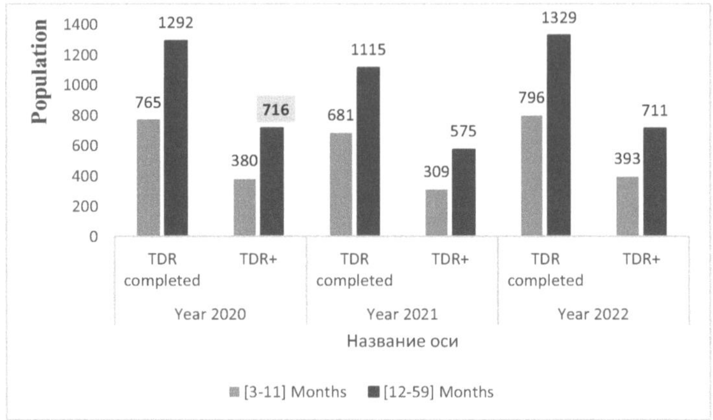

Figure 5:The number of children with a positive RDT compared to those who had an RDT during the CPS

In 2020, the number of children with a positive RDT was higher, with 716 in the [12-59] months age group.

3.2 Reasons that prevented children from taking CPS medication

Table V Reasons that prevented children from taking CPS medicines

Patterns	Average number of children seen without CPS medication					
	[3-11] months			[12-59] months		
	2020	2021	2022	2020	2021	2022
TDR+	380	309	393	716	575	711
Under cotrimoxazole	82	123	116	153	191	179
Allergy	0	1	4	0	2	3
Vomit 2 dose	78	110	100	135	167	114
Inability to swallow	4	1	1	5	2	3
Other	5	6	18	10	19	27

The main reason for not taking CPS drugs was a positive RDT, with 380 in 2020, 309 in 2021 and 393 in 2022 for [3-11] months and 716 in 2020, 575 in 2021 and 711 in 2022 for [12-59] months.

3.3 Percentage of children who received medication during the 4 CPS visits

Table VI Percentage of children who received medication during the 4 CPS visits

Targets	Age (months)	Year 2020	Year 2021	Year 2022
Number of children receiving SPAQ during 4 visits	[3-11]	14687 (59%)	17004 (67%)	18194 (69%)
	[12-59]	75117 (64%)	89895 (75%)	88653 (72%)
Expected number of children	[3-11]	24868	25561	26270
	[12-59]	117241	120194	123846

By age group, the highest percentage of children who received medication from the four passages was observed in 2021, with 75% in the [12 to 59] months age group.

3.4 Minor adverse effects

Table VII Minor adverse reactions

Minor adverse effects	Workforce		
	2020	2021	2022
Late vomiting	23	0	1
Diarrhea	26	0	0
Abdominal pain	102	0	0
Sleepiness	178	0	1

The most frequent adverse reactions were somnolence (178 cases) and abdominal pain (102 cases).

3.5 Coverage rate by health area in 2020

Table VIII Coverage rate of children by health area in 2020

Health areas	[3-11] months	[12-59] months	SPAQ children received	Expected child
BANCOUMANA	77%	77%	650	846
DABAN	71%	87%	351	497
DIAGO	134%	159%	334	249
DIALAKORODJI	89%	104%	1 987	2238
DIO GARE	54%	66%	174	319
DJOLIBA	66%	61%	1 088	1656
DOGODOUMA	90%	87%	586	649
DOMBILA	89%	88%	535	604
DOUBABOUGOU	80%	89%	347	435
FALADJE	72%	80%	580	801
FARABANA	45%	48%	69	154
FARADA	76%	125%	231	303
KABALABOUGOU	52%	48%	902	1741
KALIFABOUGOU	70%	95%	465	664
KANADJIGUILA	100%	103%	1 491	1492
KOKO 1	46%	78%	165	357
KOKO 2	24%	22%	90	377
KATI CORO	75%	80%	557	746
MALIBOUGOU	116%	143%	1 285	1112
MORIBABOUGOU	49%	84%	422	853
NANA KENIEBA	111%	108%	330	298
NEGUELA	28%	21%	166	589
NGABAKORO	50%	134%	168	333
NIOUMA MAKA	102%	108%	383	376
OUEZZINDOUGOU	76%	93%	183	239
SAFO	43%	78%	467	1094
SANANFARA	193%	89%	1 356	704
SANDAMA	165%	108%	682	413
SANGAREBOUGOU	69%	70%	1 038	1500
SIBY	77%	95%	606	783
SONIKEGNY	67%	89%	184	276
TORODO	50%	50%	266	527
YELEKEBOUGOU	82%	94%	545	662
DIO BA	103%	103%	184	179
DJIGUIDALA	65%	82%	94	144
NIAME	87%	104%	139	159
KOURSALE	101%	95%	300	298
TITIBOUGOU	74%	134%	150	201

In 2020, the highest coverage in terms of the number of children receiving all the medicines during the 4 CPS visits was observed in the [3-11] months age group in the Sananfara health area, with 193%.

3.6 Coverage rate by health area in 2021

Table IX Coverage rates by health area in 2021

Health areas	[3-11] months	[12-59] months	Expected child	Child SPAQ received
BANCOUMANA	90%	92%	869	783
DABAN	66%	91%	511	339
DIAGO	142%	108%	256	364
DIALAKORODJI	113%	142%	2300	2593
DIO GARE	78%	76%	328	257
DJOLIBA	89%	96%	1702	1512
DOGODOUMA	101%	103%	667	676
DOMBILA	92%	108%	621	570
DOUBABOUGOU	107%	98%	447	480
FALADJE	93%	101%	633	586
BASSABOUGOU	83%	85%	190	157
FARABANA	108%	84%	158	171
FARADA	117%	149%	312	366
KABALABOUGOU	68%	87%	1789	1221
KALIFABOUGOU	73%	92%	682	496
KANADJIGUILA	97%	110%	1534	1493
KOKO 1	61%	91%	367	224
KOKO 2	100%	68%	387	386
KATI CORO	88%	89%	767	674
MALIBOUGOU	101%	126%	1143	1158
MORIBABOUGOU	93%	92%	877	812
NANA KENIEBA	102%	108%	307	312
NEGUELA	95%	90%	606	577
NGABAKORO	86%	167%	342	294
NIOUMA MAKANA	76%	85%	386	294
OUEZZINDOUGOU	118%	125%	245	288
SAFO	37%	75%	1125	415
SANANFARA	98%	101%	724	712
SANDAMA	113%	116%	424	478
SANGAREBOUGOU	71%	59%	1541	1098
SIBY	90%	105%	805	727
SONIKEGNY	85%	102%	284	243
TORODO	53%	52%	542	286
YELEKEBOUGOU	111%	96%	680	752
DIO BA	102%	98%	184	188
DJIGUIDALA	81%	66%	148	119
NIAME	82%	114%	164	134
KOURSALE	99%	102%	307	305
TITIBOUGOU	63%	123%	207	130

In 2021, the highest coverage in terms of the number of children receiving all the medicines during the 4 CPS visits was observed in the [12-59] months age group in the NGABAKORO health area, at 167%.

Coverage rates by health area in 2022

Table X Coverage rate by health area in 2022

Health areas	[3-11] months	[12-59] months	Expected children	SPAQ children received
BANCOUMANA	71%	86%	893	637
DABAN	68%	73%	525	358
DIAGO	88%	98%	263	232
DIALAKORODJI	109%	111%	2364	2567
DIO GARE	84%	92%	193	162
DJOLIBA	91%	92%	1422	1294
SAMAYANA	87%	92%	327	284
DOGODOUMA	103%	99%	686	708
DOMBILA	105%	100%	638	668
DOUBABOUGOU	107%	101%	460	491
FALADJE	95%	93%	651	616
BASSABOUGOU	94%	115%	195	183
FARABANA	147%	231%	163	240
FARADA	86%	162%	172	149
KABALABOUGOU	76%	82%	1839	1404
KALIFABOUGOU	88%	94%	701	620
KANADJIGUILA	93%	100%	1416	1323
KOKO 1	65%	82%	377	244
KOKO 2	87%	74%	398	345
KATI CORO	99%	94%	788	782
MALIBOUGOU	91%	96%	997	904
MORIBABOUGOU	80%	91%	477	383
FOMBABOUGOU	51%	83%	424	216
NANA KENIEBA	109%	109%	315	343
NEGUELA	65%	62%	623	404
NGABAKORO	88%	183%	352	310
NIOUMA MAKANA	238%	140%	397	943
OUEZZINDOUGOU	106%	103%	252	268
SAFO	56%	90%	1156	650
SANANFARA	100%	100%	744	744
SANDAMA	105%	103%	436	459
SANGAREBOUGOU	93%	83%	1584	1467
SIBY	98%	99%	828	808
SONIKEGNY	71%	85%	292	208
TORODO	93%	63%	357	331
YELEKEBOUGOU	108%	103%	699	757
DIO BA	89%	100%	189	168
DJIGUIDALA	96%	95%	152	146
NIAME	82%	120%	168	138
KOURSALE	114%	114%	315	360
KAMBILA	122%	160%	148	180
MAGNAMBOUGOU	98%	100%	143	140
WADOUGOU S	160%	141%	178	285
MAMARIBOUGOU	69%	108%	160	110
TITIBOUGOU	108%	114%	213	229

In 2022, the highest coverage in terms of the number of children receiving all medicines during the 4 CPS visits was observed in the [3-11] months age group in the NIOUMA MAKANA health area, at 238%.

3.7 Incidence of malaria in children under 5 in health facilities.

Table XI Incidence of malaria in children under 5 in health facilities

Years	Incidence of malaria in children under 5 in hospitals and health facilities
2020	190,3 ‰
2021	272,3 ‰
2022	275,7 ‰

In 2022 the incidence rate was a remarkable 275.7 ‰ of cases.

COMMENTS AND DISCUSSION

IV. COMMENTS AND DISCUSSION

Limits and difficulties

At the time of data collection, information on adverse events was not available in the 2021 and 2022 reports, which is one of the limitations of this study. This evaluation only concerned the Kati health district, and therefore does not reflect that of the country as a whole.

Access to the reports from the various CPSs in the Health Information System department was not easy, given the workload of the person in charge. Our limited knowledge of the Dhis2 platform greatly slowed down the data processing process.

4.1 The number of children with a positive RDT compared to those who underwent RDT during CPS.

In our 2020 study, the number of TDR-positive children was higher in 2020, with 716 (53.28%) in the [12-59] months age group. Our results are comparable to those of **DENA P** in **2020**, which according to these results in 2019 on 303 of the numbers tested 49.8% were TDR positive [21]. On the other hand, our results are close to those of **SANOGO M** in **2020**, who in his study found that over the year 2015 the sum of positive TDRs amounted to 51.57%, 44.45% in 2016, 47.84% in 2017 and 38.84% in 2018 [22]. We can conclude that children under the age of 5 are the targets most susceptible to malaria, hence the adoption of the CPS campaign in children under 5.

4.2 Reasons that prevented children from taking CPS medication

In our study, the main reason preventing children from taking CPS drugs over the last three years was a positive RDT. Our results differ from those of **DIARRA B.M** in **2021**, who in his study found that the main reason was the unavailability of children's guardians during administration [23]. We can conclude that this is due to the fact that parents are not aware of the CPS campaign program.

4.3 Children who received medication during the 4 CPS visits

In our study by age group, the highest percentage of children who received medication in all four rounds was observed in 2021, with 75% in the 12-59 months age group. Our results are comparable to those of **MALLE A.M** in **2021**, who evaluated the number of children who received CPS medication during the four passages per year and obtained the following results: 10% at 1er Passage, 12% at 2ème Passage, 34% at 3ème passage and 44% at 4ème and last passage [24]. This increase is thought to be due to the population's adherence to the various CPS campaigns, thanks to awareness-raising by the health authorities.

4.4 Minor adverse effects

In our study, the most frequent minor adverse effects were abdominal pain with 102% of cases in 2020 and somnolence with 178% of cases. However, our results are similar to those of **CISSE B** et **Al** in **2015,** whose most frequent adverse events were digestive disorders with a majority of 83.2% [25]. These adverse effects are not new and are well reported in the summary of product characteristics (SPC).

4.5 Coverage rate by health area

Over the last three years, the number of health areas in the Kati district has risen to 38 in 2020 and 42 in 2022. The health area with the highest coverage rate of children having received all the medicines during the 4 visits for [3-11] months is the SANANFARA health area with 193% and for [12-59] months is the DIAGO health area with 159% in 2020. In 2021, the DIAGO health area recorded the highest number of children having received all the medicines during the 4 visits in the [3-11] months age group at 142%, and in the [12-59] months age group it was the NGABAKORO health area at 167%. In 2022, the NIOMA MAKANA health area led with 238% of [3-11] month-olds and 183% of [12-59] month-olds in NGABAKORO. This high participation rate was also noted by **SANOGO M** in **2020,** who determined that coverage in the Koulouba health area was 103%, while coverage in N'Tomikorobougou, Badialan and Samè was 114%, 98.89% and 96.84% respectively. However, these overruns in some of our results could be explained by the addition of a floating population, which may be holidaymakers or new district residents.

4.6 Malaria incidence rate

In our study, we found that in 2022 the incidence was remarkable with 275.7 ‰ cases. Our results are comparable to those of **KOUAKOU,** who in his study made a monthly comparison on the incidence of malaria infection of study participants having benefited or not from SPC and had found the following results: 4.3% (August); 5.1% (September); 10.7% (October); 16.5% (November) [26]. Our results are different to those of **SISSOKO M,** who had made a representative table of malaria incidence from 2013 to 2016 and had obtained the following proportions: 281.2 in 2013; 237.5 in 2014; 206.9 in 2015 and 214.3 in 2016 [27]. However, our results differ from those of **DICKO A,** who in his study compared the number of malaria cases between 2014 and 2015 in the CScoms of Kangaba and Kolokani and obtained in Kangaba a drop of 27% in 2014 and 39% in 2015; in Kolokani a drop of 21% in 2014 and

38% in 2015 [28]. This difference could be interpreted by the fact that, in his study, he had compared the number of malaria cases between 2014 and 2015, the year covered by the SPC, versus 2013, the year without the SPC.

CONCLUSION AND RECOMMENDATIONS

V. CONCLUSIONS AND RECOMMENDATIONS

Conclusions

At the end of this work, the evaluation of the data shows satisfactory SPC coverage, and a regular progression of the various passages over the last three years. The rate of RDT positivity increased each year. The main reasons for not taking the medication were positive RDTs, vomiting and children on co-trimoxazole. Minor adverse reactions were noted during the various campaigns, but no major cases. However, evaluation of data from the corresponding years shows an increase in the incidence of the disease.

It would be necessary to improve the quality of awareness of both the adverse effects of medicines and those of children's guardians.

Recommendations

At the end of this study on the analysis of data from seasonal malaria chemoprevention campaigns in children aged 3-59 months in the Kati health district over the last three years 2020-2021-2022, we made the following recommendations addressed:

To health workers

❖ Set up a system to monitor compliance with treatment, to ensure that doses are actually taken at home, and to assess the effectiveness of chemoprevention;

❖ Redouble efforts to detect and report adverse events reported by households;

❖ Strengthen communication and awareness-raising at all levels.

To the people of the Kati district

❖ Comply with personal and collective malaria prevention measures;

❖ Follow professional advice on malaria.

REFERENCES

VI. REFERENCES

1. WHO. World Malaria Report. 2022.

2. WHO. Chemoprevention of seasonal malaria by administering sullfadoxine-pyrimethamine and amodiaquine to children 2013.

3. Global Malaria Programme. Accessed: July 14, 2023. [Online]. Available at: https://www.who.int/fr/teams/global-malaria-programme/case-management/treatment.

4. Malaria (ANOFEL) Association Française des Enseignants de Parasitologie et Mycologie 2014 [Internet]. [cited 2023 Sep 6]. Available from: https://fr.readkong.com/page/paludisme-association -française-des-enseignants-de-6695706.

5. dhis2, "Système d'information sanitaire du Mali, incidence du paludisme dans le district sanitaire de Kati en 2020, 2021, 2022", january 2023.

6. PNLP: PALUDISME | Paludisme Généralités. Accessed: June 6, 2024. [Online]. Available at: https://www.pnlpcotedivoire.org/paludisme-generalites/.

7. Malaria: causes, symptoms and treatments - Health tips. Accessed: July 14, 2023. [Online]. Available at: https://www.pharma-gdd.com/fr/paludisme-causes-symtpomes-et-traitements.

8. NMCP: Medicines for the prevention and treatment of malaria: Canadian recommendations for the prevention and treatment of malaria - Canada.ca. 2019. [Cited July 14, 2023). Available at: https://www.canada.ca/fr/sante-publique/services/ccmtmv/recommandations-canadienne-prevention-traitement-paludisme-malaria/chapitre-8-medicaments.html.

9. Diagnosis of malaria: Canadian recommendations for the prevention and treatment of malaria. Accessed: July 14, 2023. [Online]. Available at: https://www.canada.ca/fr/sante-publique/services/ccmtmv/recommandations-canadienne-prevention-traitement-paludisme-malaria/chapitre-6-diagnostic-paludisme.html.

10. All about rapid testing, hiv.org. Accessed: July 14, 2023. [Online]. Available at: https://vih.org/20090928/tout-sur-les-tests-de-depistage-rapide/.

11. TEST MALARIA HRP-2, st, 1 test (STANDARD Q P.f 09MAL10D)", MSF. Accessed: June 6, 2024. [Online]. Available at: https://www.unicat.msf.org/fr/cat/product/81056.

12. G. A. B. Patrick, "Evaluation of the "SD BIOLINE Malaria Antigen Pf (HRP2; pLDH)" test for the rapid diagnosis of malaria in Abidjan (Côte d™ Ivoire) in 2014", 2014.

13. PNLP: PRISE EN CHARGE | Traitement du Paludisme . Accessed: June 6, 2024. [Online]. Available at: https://www.pnlpcotedivoire.org/traitement-du-paludisme/.

14. Malaria prevention - Centre Hospitalier Universitaire (CHU) de Toulouse. Accessed: July 14, 2023. [Online]. Available at: https://www.chu-toulouse.fr/-prevention-du-paludisme.

15. WHO General Recommendation. Seasonal malaria chemoprevention to control Plasmodium falciparum malaria in areas of high seasonal transmission in the African sahel sub-region 2012, Accessed: 1 October 2023. [Online]. Available at: https://iris.who.int/bitstream/handle/10665/337982/WHO-HTM-GMT-2012.02-fre.pdf?isAllowed=y&sequence=1.

16. World Health Organization. Chemoprevention of seasonal malaria by administering sulfadoxine-pyrimethamine and amodiaquine to children: a field guide. Geneva: World Health Organization, 2013. Accessed: July 13, 2023. [Online]. Available from: https://apps.who.int/iris/handle/10665/85727.

17. Chemoprevention of Seasonal Malaria (CPS). "Training manual", *Med. Malar. Venture MMV*, 2013.

18. CHEMOPREVENTION CAMPAIGN - PSIMALI. Accessed: July 14, 2023. [Online]. Available at: https://www.psimali.ml/2019/10/campagne-cps/.

19. Malaria Guidelines_DHMOSHPH_2019-04_FINAL_En_0.pdf. [Cited July 13, 2023]. [Internet]. Available from: https://hr.un.org/sites/hr.un.org/files/Malaria%20Guidelines_DHMOSHPH_2019-04_FINAL_Fr_0.pd.

20. GUILBERT Cécile. The chemoprevention of seasonal malaria [Internet]. [France]: université de Lille 2; 2016 [cited 11 Dec 2019]. Available from: petitedepot.univ-lille2.fr.

21. **Dena P**. Evaluation de l'effet de la chimio-prévention du paludisme saisonnier chez les enfants de 3-59 mois dans le district sanitaire de Bafoulabé. Thèse Médecine, [20M206,P80].

22 **Sanogo M dit K**. Connaissances des mères et impact de la chimio-prévention du paludisme saisonnier chez les enfants de 3 à 59 mois dans les aires de santé Koulouba, Samè, N'Tomikorobougou et Badialan de 2015 à 2018, Thèse Pharmacie. [20P07,p69].

23. **Diarra BM.** Evaluation of seasonal malaria chemoprevention coverage in the Kadiolo health district (Mali) in 2017. Thèse Médecine, [21M74,p120].

24. **Mallé AM**. Pilot study on the use of DihydroarthémisinePiperaquine in children under 10 years of age for the chemoprevention of seasonal malaria in Kenenkoun in the health district of Koulikoro, Mali. Thèse Médecine, [21M255 ,p57].

25. **Cisse B, Diallo T, Traoré D, Denou A, Coulibaly S K, Diarra A, Coulibaly B F, Bah S, Maïga A, Maïga S**. Étude des effets indésirables lies à l'administration de Sullfadoxine-

Pyrimethamine et Amodiaquine lors de la chimio prévention du paludisme saisonnier au Mali. *Rev.* Malienne Infect. Microbiol. n° 1, Art. n° 1. June 2018. Doit: 10.53597/remim.v0i1.984.

26. **Kouakou T**. Pilot study on chemoprevention of seasonal malaria in children aged 3 months to 9 years in a high-transmission area in Mali: Dangassa. Thèse Médecine, [20M48,p75].

27. Sissoko, Ba M, Diallo D, Sanogo M, Diawara S, Guindo JB, Malan K, Diallo, Sanogo, FW, Diawara, Guindo, K, and Traore, Diop. Impact of chemoprevention of seasonal malaria in children aged 3 to 59 months in the health districts of Kangaba and Kolokani between 2013 and 2015. Rev Mali Infect Microbiol 2020 Tome 15 [Internet]. Available from: https://www.sciencedirect.com/science/article/pii/S0399077X17303876.

28. Dicko A, Diallo AI, Tembine I, Dicko Y, Dara N, Sidibe Y et Al. Impact de la Chimio Prévention du Paludisme sur la Morbidité et la Mortalité des Enfants de 3-59 Mois dans le district Sanitaire de Diré Mali: Chimio prévention du paludisme à Diré. Health Sci. *Dis.* vol. 22, n° 10, Art. n° 10, Oct. 2021. [Cited July 13, 2023]. [Internet]. Available from: http://www.hsd-fmsb.org/index.php/hsd/article/view/3022.

APPENDICES

IX. APPENDICES

Inquiry form

1. CPS year: 202...
2. Malaria incidence rate: ....%
3. Number of CPS cards distributed :

➢ [3-11[Months :...............................

➢] 12-59] Month :.............................

4. Average number of children who received a dose of SP-AQ

➢ [3-11 [Month :..............................

➢] 12-59] Month :.............................

5. Average number of children who vomited and received a second dose SP-AQ

➢ [3-11[Months :..............................

➢] 12-59] Month :.............................

6. Number of RDTs produced during the SPC

➢ [3-11[Months :..............................

➢] 12-59] Month :.............................

7. Number of positive RDTs during SPC

➢ [3-11[Months :..............................

➢] 12-59] Month :.............................

8. Reasons preventing children from taking CPS medicines

➢ TDR+ :

✓ [3-11[Months :.......................

✓] 12-59] Month :.....................

➢ Under cotrimoxazole :

✓ [3-11[Months :......................

✓] 12-59] Month :.....................

➢ Allergy :

✓ [3-11[Months :......................

✓] 12-59] Month :.....................

➢ Vomit 2 dose :

✓ [3-11[Months :......................

✓] 12-59] Month :.....................

➢ Inability to swallow :

✓ [3-11[Months :......................

- ✓] 12-59] Month :....................
- ➢ Others :
- ✓ [3-11[Months :......................
- ✓] 12-59] Month :....................

9. Percentage of children who received SP-AQ during the 4 CPS visits

- ➢ [3 -11 [Month :..............................
- ➢] 12-59] Month :.............................

10. Average rate of children receiving SP-AQ for the 4 passages

Health areas	] 3-11] Month	12-59] Months

DATA SHEET

Name: Fané

First name: Fatoumata

Date and place of birth: 21/06/1999 at Kati

Telephone: 83 37 51 74

Email: fatoumatafane03@gmail.com

Thesis title: Evaluation of data from seasonal malaria chemoprevention campaigns in children aged 3 to 59 months in the Kati health district.

Academic year: 2023-2024

City of defense: Bamako

Country of origin: Mali

Depository: FMOS/FAPH Library

Area of interest:

Summary:

This was a retrospective quantitative cross-sectional study. Data were collected over a three-month period from January 1 to March 31, 2023. The aim of this study was to evaluate data from Seasonal Malaria Chemoprevention Campaigns in children aged 3 to 59 months in the Kati health district over the past three years (2020-2021-2022). The results highlight the following points:

On satisfactory SPC coverage, and a regular flow of different passages over the last three years. The rate of positive RDTs increased each year. The main reasons for not taking the medication were positive RDTs, vomiting and children on co-trimoxazole. Minor adverse events were noted during the various campaigns, but no major cases. In our study, evaluation of data from the corresponding years shows an increase in the incidence of the disease.

Key words: Chemoprevention, Seasonal malaria.

DATA SHEET

Name: Fané

First name: Fatoumata

Date and place of birth: 21/06/1999 in Kati

Telephone: 83 37 51 74

Email: fatoumatafane03@gmail.com

Thesis title: assessment data from seasonal Malaria Chemo-Prevention Campaigns in children aged 3 to 59 months in the Kati health district.

Academic year: 2023-2024

Defense city: Bamako

Contry of origine: Mali

Place of deposit: Library of the FMOS/FAPH

Sector of interest:

Abstract:

This was a retrospective cross-sectional study of quantitative nature. The collection took place over a perriod of three months from January 1 to march31, 2023. The objective of this study was to assess data from seasonal Malaria Chemo-Prevention Campaigns in children aged 3 to 59 months in the Kati health district over the past three years (2020-2021-2022).

The results highlight the following points:

On satisfactory coverage of the CPS, and a regular progress of the different passages over the last three years. The positivity rate of RDTs wich increasy each year. The main reasons for preventing medication were positive RTDs, vomiting and children on cotrimoxazole. Minor adverse effects were noted during the various campaigns but no major cases. In our study, the assessment of data from the corresponding years chows a growth in the incidence of the disease.

Keywords: Chemo Prevention, seasonal Malaria.

GALEN'S OATH

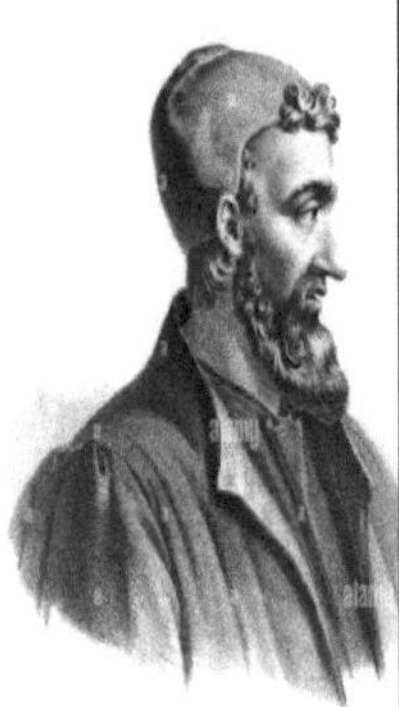

I swear, in the presence of the masters of the Faculty
of the Order of Pharmacists, and of my fellow
fellow students:
To honor those who have instructed me in the precepts
of my art, and to express my gratitude to them
by remaining faithful to their teaching,
To practice my profession conscientiously in the interest of
public health
profession with conscience and to respect not only
not only the legislation in force, but also the rules of
honor, probity and disinterestedness
disinterestedness,
Never to forget my responsibility and duties
duties towards patients and their human dignity,
Under no circumstances will I agree to use my knowledge and
knowledge and status to corrupt morals and encourage
and encourage criminal acts,
May men esteem me if I am true to my promises
faithful to my promises,
May I be covered with opprobrium and despised by my
colleagues if I fail to do so!

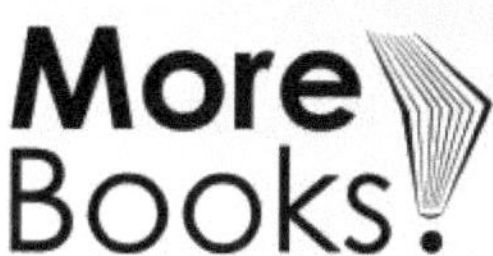

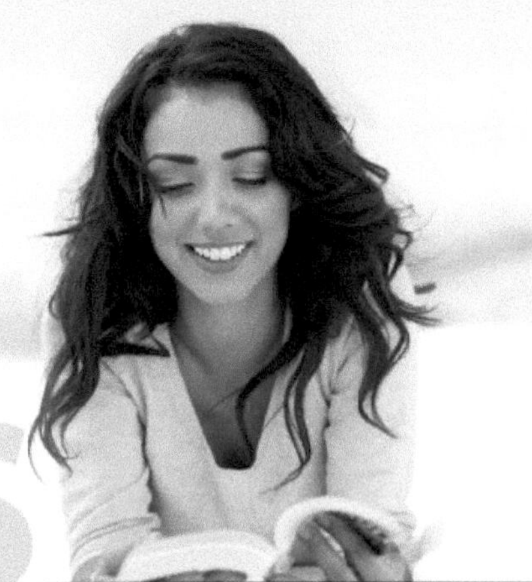

yes

I want morebooks!

Buy your books fast and straightforward online - at one of world's fastest growing online book stores! Environmentally sound due to Print-on-Demand technologies.

Buy your books online at

www.morebooks.shop

Kaufen Sie Ihre Bücher schnell und unkompliziert online – auf einer der am schnellsten wachsenden Buchhandelsplattformen weltweit! Dank Print-On-Demand umwelt- und ressourcenschonend produzi ert.

Bücher schneller online kaufen

www.morebooks.shop

info@omniscriptum.com
www.omniscriptum.com

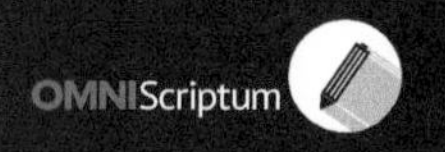

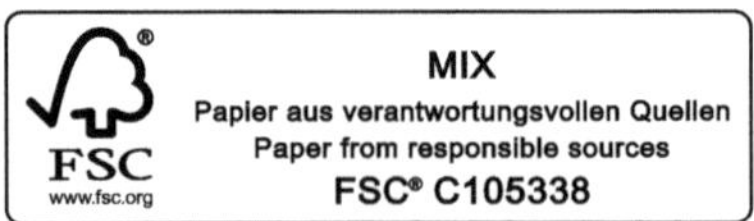

Printed by Books on Demand GmbH, Norderstedt / Germany